Love, Sex, and Menopause

Rachel Pope
Anna Myers
Jean Marino

Love, Sex, and Menopause

Dedication:

We gratefully dedicate this book to Dr. Sheryl
Kingsberg, a cherished friend and esteemed
colleague. A trailblazer in the realm of women's
sexual health, Dr. Kingsberg has pushed Female
Sexual Dysfunction to the forefront of medicine. Her
invaluable contributions, coupled with her generosity
in disseminating knowledge and serving as a guiding
mentor, have enriched us profoundly. In the words of
Sir Isaac Newton, "If I have seen further, it is by
standing on the shoulders of giants," a sentiment that
eloquently captures our deep affection and profound
gratitude for Dr. Kingsberg's inspiring presence in
our journey as practitioners.

Meet the authors:

Jean Marino: Women's Health Nurse Practitioner who is also a menopause certified provider and has a fellow designation in women's sexual health.

Anna Myers: Women's Health and Family Nurse Practitioner who is also a urology certified provider, AASECT certified sexual health counselor and has a fellow designation in women's sexual health.

Rachel Pope: Associate Professor of OB/GYN with fellowship training in global women's health, Chief of the Female Sexual Health Division at University Hospitals Cleveland Medical Center and menopause certified provider.

In 2019, Anna met Jean, a fellow Women's Health Nurse Practitioner. They hit it off and learned they had a shared interest in women's sexual health. Jean introduced Anna to the International Society for the Study of Women's Sexual Health. In 2020, Anna and Rachel met and together they formed the Female Sexual Health Division in the Urology Institute at University Hospitals Cleveland Medical Center. They invited Jean to join and they have been working closely together ever since to improve the lives of women. The three decided to start a company called "The Menopause Retreat" that offers retreats where women can talk about peri-menopause, menopause, and their sexual health in a safe space and get reliable evidenced-based information from menopause and sexual health experts. Together, they strive to create a sense of community for women to prevent the isolation that can occur during this time. Their goal is to never hear women say, "Why isn't anyone talking about menopause?"

Foreword

We want to start this book by letting you know that not all women and those who identify as women are bothered about love or sex while going through menopause. As our body and hormones change, it is actually quite natural to lose desire and interest in sex. Data backs this up. For many women, this is distressing and also causes rifts in their relationships. However, the decrease in desire for sex does not have to be a problem if it is not an issue for you. We do not need to "treat" that change if it is not bothering you. Some women also do not experience much of a change, and others experience the highest drive and best quality sex of their lives. We are all different.

This book is intended for women, who are like many of our patients and are frustrated by the changes often associated with menopause and want information about what is happening to their bodies. These women are looking to access ways to improve what symptoms are bothering them or causing discomfort. This book is **not intended** for women who do not care about sex, but their partners do and they just want to please their partner. For those women, we encourage you to seek out help from a relationship counselor or therapist. Of course, we understand the desire to make the people we love happy, but not by enduring pain or frustration.

We encourage you to take a moment to reflect before reading on because we want to empower you to live your best life.

The following chapters and topics are common issues brought up to us by our patients. We will delve into the medical aspects of menopause and the changes with sex that come up for many women. We will explore the treatments and therapies that are available to you and what our patients have told us about them.

In the appendix are several resources that we've found useful, including medications that influence libido, and a letter you can give your partner about this stage of life.

Women are smart. We trust them and we listen to them.

This book is our chance to share with you what they have taught us.

Introduction:

Menopause is normal. It is the planned end of ovarian function, meaning the planned end of ovulation and all women should be so lucky as to reach menopause. Menopause can be freeing: no more painful periods, no more worrying about bleeding, no more worrying about an unplanned pregnancy. In addition, menopause can be a time in a woman's life when she can focus on herself. Nevertheless, many women have a negative correlation with menopause. They tell us they fear menopause or are embarrassed to be menopausal. Some women at our retreats tell us they associate menopause with the words: "old," "dry," and "invisible."

What 3 words do you think of when you hear the word menopause?

1.

2.

3.

If you, too, feel negatively towards menopause or if you think sex and menopause are paradoxical, perhaps you have chosen to believe a negative story that was told to you. We want to help you change the story you are telling yourself. Because it is just that, a story. Yes, there can be bothersome menopausal symptoms and yes, you may need some assistance with products or medications; but menopause can and should be positive and you can continue or start to have a healthy sex life. And we can help!

Start by writing down 3 positive things about menopause:

1.

2.

3.

Chapter 1: Hot Flashes and Sex: Who Wants To Get Any Hotter?

Jean Marino

Kelly is 49 years old and complaining of hot flashes. She describes them as a sense of warmth that starts in her face and works up towards her scalp where she starts sweating. The hot flashes not only make her uncomfortable, but they also make her feel anxious and embarrassed by how red her face gets, and she feels less confident about her body image. Kelly is convinced everyone is noticing. She has to dress in layers and finds she has her wrap off and then on….and then off again. Kelly can only sleep with a fan on and her summer nightgown, even in the winter. At night, she finds that she has her covers off and then on…and then off again. Except for at night when he is cold in their bedroom, her husband Paul, is somewhat oblivious to her hot flashes and finds her as attractive as always. He wants to have sex with her, but Kelly tells me that she cannot imagine being that physically close to him and becoming any hotter or sweatier.

Questions to consider:

1. How would you describe your hot flashes?
   a. Not bad, I don't know what the fuss is all about.
   b. I don't like them, but I can manage and laugh about it.

c. I feel like I am in hell.

2. Do hot flashes affect how you feel about sex?
   a. No, I haven't noticed a difference.
   b. Well I'm already undressed for most of the day since I am feeling so warm; so why not just have sex?
   c. I can't imagine adding someone else's body heat to mine, stay away unless you are holding a fan.

Hot flashes, also known as night sweats or vasomotor symptoms, are one of the most common and recognizable symptoms of menopause. They can range from feeling slightly warmed or flushed to soaking sweats. Furthermore, a feeling of your heart racing or chills can accompany hot flashes. Researchers are not entirely sure what causes a hot flash but we do know that there is a disruption of temperature control caused by a narrowing of the thermoneutral zone (a person's internal thermostat), a decline in estrogen, and a change in the firing of specific nerve cells in the brain referred to as the KNDY neurons (Rance 2009). Serotonin and overall health of the brain may also influence hot flashes. Unfortunately, it is impossible to predict how long the hot flashes will last. On average women have hot flashes for 7 years but some women experience them even into their 60s and beyond (Avis et al. 2015).

The good news is that there are several treatment options for hot flashes. The gold standard is menopausal hormone therapy. Estrogen works better than anything else for treating hot flashes and you can be prescribed either estradiol or conjugated equine estrogen; they both work equally well for hot flashes. If you still have your uterus, you need to take a progestogen to protect it from the estrogen. If your uterus has been surgically removed (hysterectomy) then you only need estrogen. Menopausal hormone therapy can have a bad reputation, but it may be safer than you think. Perimenopausal women (women who have menopausal symptoms but have not gone 12 months in a row without a period) and women within 10 years of their last period and/or less than 60 years old are usually great candidates for hormone therapy.

Women with a history of hormone dependent cancer, such as breast cancer or uterine cancer, are not good candidates for systemic hormone therapy-meaning the hormones would get to the entire body which is different from most vaginal hormone therapy. In addition, women with a history of a blood clot in their chest, arm, or leg; women at high risk of heart disease, or women with a history of liver or gallbladder disease are most likely not good candidates for systemic hormone therapy. The 2022 Menopause Society position statement on hormone therapy is a great resource regarding safety and risk and is available online.

Other options for treatment of hot flashes include prescriptions that are not hormones. There are currently two non-hormonal prescriptions that are approved by the Federal Drug Administration (FDA) for the treatment of hot flashes, Brisdelle and Veozah. Brisdelle treats hot flashes by increasing the available amount of serotonin and it has a side effect of drowsiness that may help women sleep. Veozah is a medication that targets the KNDY neurons that influence a persons' internal thermostat to decrease hot flashes.

Other medications can be prescribed that are off label, meaning they have not been FDA approved for hot flashes, but studies have shown they are safe and effective for the treatment of hot flashes. Options include a selective serotonin reuptake inhibitor (SSRI) or a serotonin and norepinephrine reuptake inhibitor (SNRI), medications usually prescribed for mood changes such as anxiety or depression, but they also help with hot flashes, most likely due to the role of serotonin in hot flashes. Potential side effects may include weight gain, a decrease in sex drive, or difficulty reaching orgasm. Gabapentin is a medication often used for nerve pain but can be prescribed for hot flashes. Potential side effects include drowsiness and weight gain. Lastly, Oxybutynin is a medication often used for overactive bladder but is helpful in treating hot flashes. The most common side effects are dry mouth and constipation.

13

There are several medications that you can purchase without a prescription; however, since they are not regulated by the FDA, the formulas are not standardized and therefore the research is limited and difficult to generalize. Keep in mind that just because a medication, herb, or supplement does not require a prescription, it does not guarantee it is safer than a prescription option.

Of the options for behavioral modifications, cognitive behavioral therapy (CBT) has the most evidence to support it for the treatment of hot flashes. A provider trained in CBT can help you change your expectations and thoughts to cope with hot flashes. CBT doesn't decrease hot flashes, but research has shown that it still improves women's quality of life.

Back to Kelly:

Kelly chose menopausal hormone therapy. Not only did her hot flashes lessen, but also her moods felt better, and she slept better. Kelly found that she was much more interested in sex once her menopausal symptoms improved and she felt more like her "old self." And she didn't mind getting sweaty if it was during sexual play.

In summary, hot flashes are common, they can be mild or severe, and it is unpredictable for how long they will last. The good news is that they will eventually get better or at least less intense and frequent. Keep in mind that you have several options for treatment and you do not have to suffer. If hot flashes are decreasing your quality of life, including limiting sexual play, please consider treatment.

Positive affirmation: I will continue to love and respect my body, I am always enough.

References:

Rance NE. Menopause and the human hypothalamus: evidence for the role of kisspeptin/neurokinin B neurons in the regulation of estrogen negative feedback. Peptides. 2009 Jan;30(1):111-22.

Avis NE, Crawford SL, Greendale G, Bromberger JT, Everson-Rose SA, Gold EB, Hess R, Joffe H, Kravitz HM, Tepper PG, Thurston RC; Study of Women's Health Across the Nation. Duration of menopausal vasomotor symptoms over the menopause transition. JAMA Intern Med. 2015 Apr;175(4):531-9.

The Menopause Society. The 2022 hormone therapy position statement of the North American Menopause Society. *Menopause.* 202229(7); 767-794.

Chapter 2. My Vagina F'ing Hurts!

Rachel Pope

"It just hurts so much during and throbs with pain after," Anne told me. She explained that sex was always an important part of her relationship with her husband, equally for both of them. She wanted to continue having vaginal penetrative intercourse and continue the intimacy that it brought them. She told me that her desire has decreased, but she's not sure if that's menopause or because of the pain.

"Probably a little of both," I told her. I recalled one of my mentors Dr. Andrew Goldstein saying, "Who would want to walk on broken glass?"

Questions to consider:

1. Have you experienced pain with sex?
   a. Only the first time I had sex.
   b. Occasionally if I'm not really "feeling the mood."
   c. Isn't sex always painful for women?

2. Have you looked at your vulva, vestibule or vagina recently?
   a. Never, I do not want to see any of it!
   b. Once while delivering my baby.
   c. I regularly look with a mirror.

When sex begins to hurt, it loses its appeal. If you are unaware of how to reduce the pain, you might decide that intimacy is gone.

I told her that I would like to examine her first so that I can assess the physical aspect of where the pain is coming from, but I told her I could already guess two things based on her story. The first, is that she describes the pain from the very beginning with penetration, which tells me that there's been some vaginal narrowing, a common attribute of menopause. The second is that she describes a soreness or rug burn feeling afterwards, which tells me she's not lubricated enough.

If a person is feeling pain with vaginal sex from the point of penetration, her body is going to stop the process of arousal which causes lubrication. Not only that, without as much estrogen in her vaginal tissues due to menopause, she does not have the same baseline moisture in the vaginal tissues. Therefore, the friction of vaginal intercourse is literally going to be more friction than is pleasurable. There are many lubricants available to help with this, but not all are equal. A silicone-based lubricant is going to provide more protection to her vaginal tissues and will ease some of that. A regular vulvar moisturizer may also be necessary to supplement the overall moisture that will make things comfortable. The most important thing, however, is vaginal estrogen.

Vaginal estrogen is a key element to a healthy vagina. Estrogen keeps the environment of the vagina acidic, which keeps the bacteria burden low (or at least low enough as to not cause a urinary tract infection). It also improves healthy blood supply to the tissues, which helps with moisture and natural lubrication. This moisture in turn, contributes to the "stretchiness" of the tissue. After menopause, we lose the estrogen in the vagina, therefore, to improve symptoms of genitourinary syndrome of menopause (GSM– formerly known as vaginal atrophy), we prescribe a synthetic estrogen to apply vaginally. This prescription estrogen can be a cream, tablet, ring, or suppository.

I did an exam and confirmed the findings I was suspecting and made sure there were not any other signs of dermatological conditions or vulvodynia (specific pain to the labia or entrance of the vagina sometimes caused by hormonal changes or other conditions). Her anatomy was otherwise normal, but her vaginal tissues were pale and dry, exactly as expected.

There was just a small amount of vaginal narrowing, so we talked about vaginal dilation. Vaginal dilators come in different sizes and materials, but I like the silicone ones because they are a bit more gentle, but still firm. Depending on the extent of narrowing, you can purchase one which will help gently stretch the vaginal opening and help the muscles relax so that penetration is not what stretches the tissue. If narrowing is more significant, a dilator set or vaginal trainer, which starts with a small size and incrementally gets larger would work better to gradually stretch the tissue instead.

Anne is looking at me with wide eyes when I tell her about the dilators. "I know it might seem like a lot," I tell her.

"I just don't know why I have to do so much, just to have sex."

We talk a bit about men needing medications like Viagra or Cialis. We discuss the fact that humans are living so much longer and healthier than before and sex continues to be an important part of life for many of us. We chat a little about ways to make the dilating feel less of a chore. I usually recommend putting on a show you've been wanting to watch and get comfortable on your bed. Some women prefer to use it in the shower, which works too.

Positive affirmation: My pleasure is important and I'm worth pursuing it.

Chapter 3: For the Single Ladies

Rachel Pope

Tonya had been single for about five years. Unfortunately, she fell out of love with her husband of 15 years and decided she would rather be alone than unhappy. This did not mean, however, that she did not want intimacy or sex. To the contrary, she was excited to meet new people and embark on new sexual experiences. She was not looking for commitment per se, just a decent guy and a fun time. She found herself frustrated by all her friends and family around her who kept trying to make her live otherwise.

After some fun and some frustration, she decided to stop looking. She was not ready for anything serious but even the men who were on the same page as her were fraught with flaws.

While taking this intentional "break," her friends started trying to set her up with people. They all had a single male friend or co-worker they thought would be perfect. However, the only thing she had in common with these men was that they were both single.

Question to Consider:

How do you feel about being single?
  a. Great, I love all the "me time."
  b. It's ok, but maybe I do want to find someone someday.
  c. I'm disappointed, I didn't think this would be what my future looked like.

What are three things you like about being single?

1.

_____

2.

_____

3.

_____

Tonya tried to ignore the prompts from her family and friends, but she started to worry that her vagina was going to "close up" if she did not use it. While her waistline and wrinkles were expanding, she began to find it difficult to accept anything beautiful or powerful about this stage of life. She found herself envious of the older couples she knew who were active in their retirement traveling together, arm-in-arm, keeping each other engaged and healthy and experiencing the growing/changing of each other and their families together.

She came to my office to ask me what she should do during this time. We spent a while venting about ageism in our country and talked about all the positives of being single—the freedom, the ability to spend her time and her days as wanted. She asked about what to do to keep her vaginal and vulvar tissue healthy in the case of a future romance or partner. I told her, "Look, this is for you, and I don't want you to think of this as for anyone else but for you. You deserve to feel good and you probably will release some endorphins while doing it," I grabbed a brochure from my preferred company.

A vibrator. No joke. You do not need a partner to orgasm. It's healthy for women to spend time with themselves pleasuring themselves and it's a great way to relieve stress. There are so many changes as we age, but the nerves in the clitoris that respond to vibration age the slowest. Keeping the clitoral nerves sensitive is probably also a good thing and vibration should help with that. Not everyone enjoys vaginal penetration, but if you want that to be part of your intimacy in the future, get a vibrator that has that option. As we go through menopause, vaginal narrowing at the entrance of the vagina is very common. Gentle stretching with a vibrator will help reduce future pain with penetration.

A vulvar balm. We all spend so much money on moisturizers for our face and yet most women neglect their vulvas. Keep the skin of your vulva moisturized using fragrance free balms.

Vaginal estrogen. As our circulating estrogen decreases, we lose our natural vaginal estrogen supply as well. Estrogen is important for the blood supply to the tissue, to keep it soft and stretchy. Without it, the tissue becomes dry and stiff. You do not need this just for sex, but for your bladder health and often for comfort, too.

I emphasized at the end of our visit, "Remember, this is for you. If you decide to share this joy with someone else that would be great, but there's no reason to miss out on it now."

Positive Affirmation: I deserve a good life and good orgasms.

Chapter 4. Lost in Desire-Land: A Map Back to
Passion Plaza

Anna Myers

Beth initially sought my help for urinary issues. However, her attention shifted when she discovered a section about desire on my intake form. Excitedly, she expressed a desire to delve deeper into that topic than the urinary issues that brought her in. "I had no idea there were specialists for this or that I could even talk about it," she exclaimed. Over the past five years, she noticed a steady decline in her desire, which was now at an all-time low. This frustrated her, particularly because her partner still maintained a fairly robust sex drive. She wanted that level of desire as well. Beth and her partner had been together for 15 years, a second marriage for both, blending their families together. Now with the kids out of the house and a thriving consulting business they started together, she couldn't understand why her desire for intimacy had dwindled. She felt let down by her body, recalling that their last intimate encounter a few months prior was uncomfortable, arousal was slow to come, and orgasm was anything but guaranteed.

We started by examining the physical aspects, acknowledging that pain can significantly dull desire.

As a mentor once explained to me, if you touch a hot stove and get burned, your brain tells you not to do it again. The same goes for sex; if it's painful or uncomfortable, our brains say 'no thank you.' So, we promptly got Beth started on estrogen vaginal cream, and introduced her to vaginal lubricants and moisturizers. Next, we shifted our focus to arousal.

Many women come to me with low desire, and I always take time to explain what to expect from our changing bodies and what a normal sexual response looks like before suggesting any treatments. Sex education in schools often misses the mark, covering sexually transmitted infections and a basic version of the sexual response cycle, but it hardly resonates with a 50-year-old woman with a lifetime of sexual experiences. Masters and Johnson's early work on the sexual response cycle, although groundbreaking, set a standard that many women find themselves comparing to: spontaneous excitement, plateau, orgasm, and resolution.

Does this ring a bell? Fortunately, Dr. Mary Basson, a psychiatrist and professor at the University of British Columbia, recognized the need for a more nuanced understanding of sexual response, particularly for women in long-term relationships. She felt that sexual response was actually more of a cycle of overlapping phases influenced by mental and physical factors. She proposed that women might not experience spontaneous desire but might initiate sex for intimacy or to express love, becoming aroused and desiring sex after physical contact has begun—what is now known as responsive desire.

Spontaneous desire is what we often see as the gold standard that we compare ourselves to. However, women typically feel this, "spontaneous desire," in a new relationship or perhaps at a certain point in their menstrual cycle. Six months into a new relationship and that spontaneous desire is not so evident.

Mary Basson didn't take credit for this idea because other researchers had already realized this, but she did create a model that was published in 2001 to explain it. Her research normalized this for women instead of it being solely a medical condition to have a lack of spontaneous sexual desire and her model has changed how we treat women, educate women, and intervene with sexual difficulties.

So, what does all this mean for you? Use this knowledge to your advantage! Arousal can precede desire; you can become physically excited and then desire intercourse. As a colleague once put it, it's like getting on a treadmill, and then remembering, "Oh, I do enjoy this!" But what exactly turns you on?

Identifying your accelerators and brakes is power. Consider using a clitoral stimulator a few minutes before anticipated activity to jumpstart arousal, a task that might take a partner much longer to accomplish, and that's only if they know exactly what to do. Be open to experimenting with aids such as sexual tools such as vibrators, clitoral stimulators, or even watching a romantic movie—it just takes a bit of planning.

Questions to Consider:

1. What is your sexual response like?
   a. I'm the one with all the desire!
   b. I'm reluctant at first but I have an open mind. Once I'm "turned on" and experiencing arousal, I find myself enjoying and wanting intimacy with my partner.
   c. I never want intimacy. My partner complains about it. I feel guilty for not wanting to.

2. How do you and your partner feel about incorporating tools into your sexual activities in a way that is comfortable and enjoyable for both of you?
   a. I am open to buying any new device, show me the catalog.
   b. If a particular device was suggested by my healthcare provider, I would consider it.

c. I am not comfortable with any sexual aides, I don't care if they are pink or not.

3. Are there any parts of your body that you have negative conversations in your mind about that may potentially affect your confidence?
   a. I walk around naked in front of my partner.
   b. I am quick to grab a towel after getting out of the shower.
   c. I'm only naked if the lights are off and the shades are down; he can find me by following my voice.

4. List 3 body parts **you love** about yourself.

   a.
   b.
   c.

How else does that powerful sex organ, the mind, sabotage our efforts? What we let our minds tell us can hinder our desire as well. Body image is often something we shrug off, denying that we have a problem with it. We might think, "Of course I want to lose a few pounds, doesn't everyone?"

However, research in the Journal of Sexual Medicine shows that various aspects of body image, including concerns about weight, physical condition, perceived sexual attractiveness, and thoughts about the body during sexual activity, are predictors of sexual satisfaction in women (Pujols et al., 2010). Whether it's a belly, a scar from a previous surgery, or something else entirely, we all view our bodies differently.

Women struggling with poor body image are less likely to initiate sex and less likely to enjoy it. For instance, have you ever preferred making love with the lights off or felt anxious about your partner seeing certain parts of your body?

How do we change this internal dialogue? Cognitive-behavioral therapy (CBT) is a type of talk therapy that helps individuals identify and change negative thoughts and behaviors and can be helpful for women with low sexual desire. Additionally, engage in activities that make you feel sexy—whether that's a hot bath, wearing something that boosts your confidence, or indulging in self-care practices like a mani-pedi, a facial, or massage. Do something that makes you feel good about yourself.

Challenge yourself to replace negative thoughts with positive affirmations about parts of your body that you appreciate and make you feel attractive.

Remember, the person beside you is there because they want to be, despite any insecurities or hang ups you might have about yourself. They likely don't share the same concerns.

Below are a few additional strategies I often discuss with my patients:

Embrace Mindfulness: Stay present and non-judgmental in the moment. Remember, you can't fully experience and critique ourselves simultaneously. As women, we often try to play and be a spectator at the same time. Worrying about your partner's experience or how your body looks only detracts from your experience, it does not add to it. Research has shown that mindfulness practices can enhance sexual desire, arousal, and orgasm (Brotto & Basson, 2014).

Communicate: Discuss your sexual desires and needs with your partner to foster a more satisfying sexual experience for both of you. Studies have shown that increased sexual communication correlates with higher orgasm frequency in women and greater relationship and sexual satisfaction in both partners (Journal of Marital & Family Therapy, 2017).

Variety is the Spice of Life: Experimenting with different sexual activities, positions, and even genital vibratory tools can heighten satisfaction. Guess et al., 2017 found that genital vibratory stimulation device use resulted in uniform improvements in sexual function, satisfaction, sexually related distress and genital sensation.

Prioritize Your Health: Maintain a balanced diet, get regular exercise, and ensure you're getting enough sleep—all of which contribute to a healthy sexual desire (Kalmbach et al., 2015).

Take Care of Your Mental Health: Don't overlook the impact of psychological factors such as stress, anxiety, and depression on your sexual desire and your willingness to seek treatment for low desire.

Now, back to Beth. She returned for her follow-up appointment, eager to share her progress. After our last session, she and her partner had a heart-to-heart and decided to purchase one of the sexual tools we discussed. She happily reported no more issues with dryness, pain, or desire; in fact, she was fully aroused by the time they engaged in penetrative sex. To her delight, her partner was turned on by her using the device.

Affirmation: I'm enough, I'm beautiful and desirable just the way I am.

References:

Brotto LA, Basson R. Group mindfulness-based therapy significantly improves sexual desire in women. Behav Res Ther. 2014 Jun;57:43-54. doi: 10.1016/j.brat.2014.04.001. Epub 2014 Apr 18. PMID: 24814472.

Guess MK, Connell KA, Chudnoff S, Adekoya O, Richmond C, Nixon KE, Freeman K, Melman A. The Effects of a Genital Vibratory Stimulation Device on Sexual Function and Genital Sensation. Female Pelvic Med Reconstr Surg. 2017 Jul-Aug;23(4):256-262. doi: 10.1097/SPV.0000000000000357. PMID: 27918337.

Hartmann U, Philippsohn S, Heiser K, Rüffer-Hesse C. Low sexual desire in midlife and older women: personality factors, psychosocial development, present sexuality. Menopause. 2004 Nov-Dec;11(6 Pt 2):726-40.

Kalmbach DA, Arnedt JT, Pillai V, and Ciesla JA. The impact of sleep on female sexual response and behavior: A pilot study. J Sex Med 2015;12:1221–1232.

Pujols Y, Meston CM, and Seal BN. The association between sexual satisfaction and body image in women. J Sex Med 2010;7:905–916.

Chapter 5. Low Desire: I want to want to…

Rachel Pope

"It's too much work. I'm done. I am putting in so much effort and she isn't doing anything."

I was seeing my patient, Jennifer, back for follow up. She had been doing well. She was using vaginal estrogen to help with improve the dryness of her vaginal tissues, and no longer needed to use her vaginal dilator because she had already made the improvements to her pelvic floor muscles to prevent pain with sex.

Many women develop tightened pelvic floor muscles that can be from stress or other pain syndromes like endometriosis or recurrent urinary tract infections, among other causes. This creates a tension response in the pelvic floor muscles resulting in trigger points. Just as we can develop trigger points in our shoulders or back, we can develop them in our pelvic floor, and they can cause a tremendous amount of pain when not addressed. A pelvic floor physical therapist can help assess for this type of pain and guide a person through treatment and prevention. Sometimes injections or vaginal medications are recommended. Sometimes a pelvic wand or vaginal dilator is recommended by health care providers or pelvic floor physical therapists. Regardless, treatment of pelvic pain including vaginal changes with menopause can be time consuming.

Question to consider:

1. Have you had to put in effort to maintain your sex life?
    a. No effort, it all comes easily to me.
    b. I do need to use a lubricant, but that's about it.
    c. I need the right music, the right lighting, and the right scented candles.

Even without her pelvic floor exercises, Jennifer was spending a significant amount of time each week either taking a medication or applying a medicated cream. She had just started systemic testosterone daily for desire. She really was putting in a lot of effort. I affirmed that fact for her and empathized with the feeling that her partner was not putting much effort into any part of their relationship.

She opened up a bit more, "I just don't have any interest."

The most difficult thing is to convince yourself to do something about a problem you don't feel motivated to fix. If you are not interested in sex, it takes a lot of energy to choose to see a healthcare provider and start a prescription medication or treatment.

"What would you like to do?" I asked her.

"To just not have to do anything extra to be 'normal,'" she said.

I understood this sentiment and honestly, many of my patients feel this way, whether they have low desire, overactive bladder, or pelvic pain. It feels like an arduous chore to take medications, spend the money and time on healthcare for things that you feel like should come easily or used to come easily.

I told her I understood that and that maybe it would be good to have this conversation with her partner.

"Listen," I told her, "There are other medications for desire, and testosterone might be a good option for you, but none of it is going to be worth it if you and your partner aren't on the same page. Even if this is something you are doing for yourself, not just for the sake of the relationship, you need to know that the other person is there for you."

I asked her if she'd be open to seeing a behavioral health specialist who focuses on sexuality and couples. She said yes, so that's what she did. It's not always easy to convince my patients to see a behavioral health specialist or therapist, but most are happy once they do.

Positive Affirmation: I deserve all the happiness and it can be available to me.

Chapter 6. Low Libido and Medications-How to Get Motivated

Jean Marino

Stephanie is 55 years old and in a long-term relationship with whom she considers her best friend. Unfortunately, their sex life is more reflective of two friends instead of two lovers. Stephanie used to have a relatively high drive for sex but now she has lost almost all interest. She doesn't have any pain with sexual play, no negative associations with sex, and she can reach orgasm, but the drive has vanished. Even though she has a great relationship, her low to absent libido is causing strain. Her partner is taking it personally and she is feeling guilty.

Questions to consider:

1. How is your sex drive?
   a. High, even after all this time I still want sex with my partner.
   b. Moderate, I might not be thinking about it, but once we get going, I'm onboard.
   c. Low/none, I would much rather watch Netflix.

2. How do you feel about medication for your sex drive?
   a. I don't need it, life is good.
   b. I would be worried about side effects and safety.

c. Yes please, I need help.

Numerous factors influence sex drive or libido. Sometimes the factors are physical: pain with sexual play, difficulty reaching orgasm, or low arousal/lubrication. Sometimes it is more psychological: history of trauma, negative association with sex, problems within the relationship, anxiety or depression. It may be due to medications, the most common being medications for both anxiety and depression. Furthermore, if you are having bothersome symptoms of menopause: hot flashes, fatigue, difficulty sleeping, mood changes, or joint pain; your desire for sex could be decreased. However, for others none of the aforementioned factors are relevant, but there is still low desire. Keep in mind that low sex drive is only a problem if it bothers you and you would like treatment. Sometimes women "want to want."

The good news is that there are prescription medications for the treatment of low sex drive in women. The diagnostic term is: "Hypoactive Sexual Desire Disorder." Flibanserin came to the market in 2015 and was the first FDA approved medication for low desire in premenopausal women. It was studied and proven safe and effective in menopausal women, but the FDA only approved it for premenopausal women. Therefore, its use in menopausal women is "off label," meaning there is information that it is safe and effective but it is not FDA approved.

Flibanserin increases both dopamine and Norethindrone, hormones in the brain that improve desire. It is recommended to take it at bedtime because the most likely side effect is drowsiness or dizziness. Other side effects may include improved mood or weight loss. The increase in drive is not immediate; you may start to notice that you don't mind if your partner initiates sexual play and then eventually you may find that you are thinking about sex. Therefore, Flibanserin should be taken for 8-12 weeks to determine if it is effective.

A second option is Bremelanotide which was FDA approved in 2019. Instead of the gradual increase in desire with Flibanserin, Bremelanotide is an injection you would administer to yourself that would start to work within 45 minutes and lasts for approximately 16 hours. This medication also increases dopamine to improve desire but it also has a physical effect: increased arousal, lubrication, and orgasm. You may notice that you physically feel "turned on." The most common side effects are facial flushing and nausea. The recommendation is to administer Bremelanotide 1-2 times/week, which makes it a nice option for women who do not want to be on medication continually and prefer to plan their date nights.

A third option is testosterone; a hormone naturally found in women but does decrease with age. Testosterone is not FDA approved for women but does have research to support its use for improving low desire in menopausal women; this is another example of an "off label use." The goal of testosterone therapy should not be to give women high amounts of testosterone, but rather keep the testosterone levels within normal range for women, but increased. Therefore, blood work is very important not only prior to starting treatment, but periodically during treatment. If testosterone levels stay within normal limits, side effects should be minimal to none. You may start to notice an improvement within 4-6 weeks and pending your labs and response, the dosing may be adjusted. However, by 6 months if you have not noticed any improvement then testosterone may not be the right choice.

There are numerous supplements and medications that are for purchase without a prescription. Unfortunately, since they are not regulated by the FDA, the formulas are not standardized, research is limited, and results are difficult to generalize.

Back to Stephanie. After reviewing the prescription options for treatment of low desire in women, Stephanie ultimately chose Flibanserin. She liked the idea of spontaneous desire and the side effects of a better night's sleep, improved mood, and weight loss were appealing. After the first 1-2 months, she wasn't sure if her desire was improving, but at her 3 month follow up appointment she noticed that her desire had improved. Stephanie was also sleeping better and lost 3 pounds which she thought may have also improved her desire for sex. Both she and her partner were happy with the improved intimacy, something they had both missed.

In summary, there are numerous reasons for a woman to have low desire, but there are also treatment options. Flibanserin and testosterone may offer more spontaneous desire and Bremelanotide is designed for on demand use. Testosterone and bremelanotide may also have physical effects in addition to the desire in the brain; while flibanserin is only affecting desire in the brain. If you decide to try a prescription medication and it doesn't work, you have other options. Consider discussing your options with a healthcare provider to determine what is the best fit for you.

Positive Affirmation: I am grateful for my body and the sexual pleasure it provides me.

Chapter 7. Is My Vulva Normal?

Rachel Pope

My new patient, Lynn, was extremely nervous, according to my nurse partner who typically checks in my patients while I review their intake forms. The woman coming to see me for the first time was not forthcoming even in her intake form about why she was here except maybe to have a pap smear.

I tried to give her my warmest and most disarming smile and introduction and soon learned about a traumatic pap smear she had about a decade ago. It was so bad that she had not returned to any women's health provider or gynecologist.

She told me that she knows her genitalia is not "normal," and maybe that is why it was so painful. She wanted to know if there was any way she could do a self-pap smear or if I had other ideas to make it less painful. I asked her what she meant about her body not being normal. She said that years ago she had vaginal discharge that she thought was an infection. She went to the emergency room for evaluation and an emergency medicine physician examined her and asked her if her vulva "always looks like that."

Question to Consider:

Do you have a sense of how your vulva characteristics might compare to others?

    a. I know there are many different vulvas out there.
    b. I have no idea what my vulva even looks like.
    c. I love my vulva!

He was not specific about what he meant by the comment, and she was too mortified to ask. She left the emergency room afterwards and sobbed in the car, unwilling to tell her husband what had happened. She looked online and in pornographic images of vulvas comparing herself in a mirror to try to understand what was different and she was, "horrified." Years later, she asked her gynecologist how common it is for other women to have a vulva like hers and he told her, "Very few."

I was not sure what to expect from her exam. I thought maybe she would have very long labia, maybe she has varicose veins, or maybe something I have never seen before perhaps. When I returned to the room to examine her and sat down to examine her, I told her, "Listen, you are 100% normal!"

Her labia were not particularly long or short. Her labia majora was normal. Her clitoral glans and the prepuce (the hood that hangs over the clitoris) was normal. Her urethra was normal, her vaginal opening or introitus was normal. Her entire examination was completely within the spectrum of normal anatomy.

It dawned on me that I have probably seen over 5,000 vulvas between medical school, residency, fellowship, and in my career as a gynecologist thus far. Women otherwise really do not see each other's vulvas and the vulvas that a person might see in pornography tends to be one "type," of vulva with very short or no labia minora. Unlike men, we don't really see each other's genitalia in the gym locker room and we have to do yoga positions with a mirror to get a good look at our own. So how would any woman who is not in the medical field know what "normal" is. How powerful it is for a medical professional to tell a woman that her vulva is abnormal and for her to believe him and then go on to hate her own body for decades.

There is not one normal when it comes to our anatomy. Our vulvas, just like our faces, have common parts but are slightly different from one person to the next. I now try to remind myself to tell all my patients how normal their anatomy looks when I examine them.

Positive Affirmation:

My vulva is unique and beautiful. It is a powerful part of me!

Chapter 8: Let's Talk About (Sex) Baby: Navigating the Intimacy Iceberg

Anna Myers

Angela found herself grappling with a delicate issue in her 25-year relationship with her partner, Brad. As a nurse in her 20s, she had crossed paths with Brad, a budding entrepreneur in the insurance sector. The couple had enjoyed a robust intimate life, but recently, things had taken a turn. Brad's interest in sex had waned, leaving Angela puzzled and concerned.

Initially, Angela attributed this change to Brad's work-related stress, as he had recently expanded his business services but was short-staffed. His return home would be marked by exhaustion and irritability. However, Angela soon found herself internalizing the problem, questioning whether changes in her appearance due to menopause or the potential presence of a younger, more attractive rival had led to this issue. When Brad began experiencing difficulties maintaining an erection, and eventually was unable to achieve one at all, Angela's concerns deepened, extending beyond their relationship to Brad's overall health.

Addressing a partner's health, especially in matters of intimacy, is never a straightforward task for women or men. I've seen countless patients navigating this challenge, often expressing concern for their spouses and wondering how to get them to come in to see a medical professional. They wonder, "How do I bring it up?"

Nothing hurts someone's self-esteem like telling them they don't measure up in bed. How could a person broach the topic without damaging their partner's self-esteem? One approach I recommend is bringing your partner to your medical appointment. I love seeing the moment of realization when a partner witnesses the effort and care the other has put into their relationship. It can be an eye-opening experience, encouraging them to take an active role in finding the solution to their problem.

Angela and Brad, eager to resolve the issue, were relieved to discover that Brad's testosterone levels were significantly low. Testosterone therapy marked the turning point for Brad, revitalizing his mood, energy levels, and interest in exercise, not to mention their sex life. His cholesterol and blood pressure were normal, and there were no signs of diabetes. However, it's worth noting that these initial tests can sometimes unveil other underlying health issues, potentially life-saving discoveries. Issues affecting the blood vessels in the penis can indicate broader circulatory system problems, including potential heart issues. Addressing sexual health concerns can, in fact, be a critical step in safeguarding your male partner's overall health.

This is a gentle conversation. Approaching this topic requires sensitivity; nothing undermines a partner's confidence quite like perceived criticism of their sexual performance. Communicating with compassion and care is paramount. Talking about sexual difficulties is a challenging conversation for all couples, yet it's a crucial part of maintaining a healthy and fulfilling sexual relationship. Remember, it's not if you are going to have sexual difficulties, but when. We all have difficulties from time to time. It may be your partner now, but it might be you later.

To facilitate these conversations, consider the following strategies:

Prepare a script: "I read that heart health issues can impact erections. Maybe a doctor's appointment is in order?"

Choose the right setting: Discussing sexual issues *outside the bedroom* can create a more relaxed atmosphere.

Use "I" statements: This approach prevents blame and focuses on your feelings and experiences.

Practice active listening: Provide validation and support, creating a safe space for vulnerability.

Be open to experimentation: Explore new positions, incorporate sexual tools (toys/props), or types of sexual activity to enhance your sex life.

Research underscores the positive correlation between sexual communication and various aspects of sexual function including desire, arousal, lubrication, orgasm and erectile function. (Journal of Sex Research, 2019, Mallory et. al). Proactive couples that discuss these issues are more likely to seek and find solutions.

Questions to Consider:

1. How comfortable are you discussing sexual health with your partner?
   a. Very comfortable; we can discuss anything.
   b. I'd like to, but I don't know how.

c. I would never discuss our sex life with my partner.

2. Lack of communication about addressing sexual health issues can impact the overall health of a relationship. How do you feel about addressing these issues if they would occur with your partner?

    a. We go on regular date nights and talk about intimacy, we text throughout the week, flirting about our intimacy. We look for solutions together.
    b. It is a touchy subject, I brought it up, but it didn't go so well. I'm going to try again.
    c. I'm frustrated with my partner that I do all the work in addressing these issues.

3. Which strategies did you find helpful in overcoming the challenge of bringing up the topic of sexual difficulties with your partner?

_____

_____

_____

_____

Affirmation: I feel closer to my partner every day.

References:

Jones AC, Robinson WD, Seedall RB. The Role of Sexual Communication in Couples' Sexual Outcomes: A Dyadic Path Analysis. J Marital Fam Ther. 2018 Oct;44(4):606-623. doi: 10.1111/jmft.12282. Epub 2017 Oct 16. PMID: 29044661.

Mallory AB, Stanton AM, Handy AB. Couples' Sexual Communication and Dimensions of Sexual Function: A Meta-Analysis. J Sex Res. 2019 Sep;56(7):882-898. doi: 10.1080/00224499.2019.1568375. Epub 2019 Feb 19. PMID: 30777780; PMCID: PMC6699928.

Chapter 9. Ageism in America

Rachel Pope

Dianne came to see me as a new patient and brought a list of the treatments she had been getting from an out of state physician who runs a "fountain of youth clinic." She said that she was using so many different treatments, she thought something was working but she was not sure what. She was using transdermal progesterone, a medication I used myself when I was going through invitro fertilization (IVF) but was given to me by injection. I did some research on the transdermal route. It appeared from what I found that we cannot even metabolize this version of it. So, it definitely wasn't doing anything the way she was told to use it. Then, she showed me transdermal DHEA, and I wondered why she would need that. We use DHEA vaginally for genitourinary syndrome of menopause (GSM). It is a steroid precursor for testosterone and estrogen, so I wasn't shocked by a topical form of it, but just didn't understand why it would be used topically on the arm and not vaginally. She wasn't sure either.

The estrogen she was on made sense although we weren't sure exactly what her dose was. The problem with some of the compounded "bio-identicals" is that there's no guarantee what the dose is in each portion. The term, "bio-identical" is also misleading as it implies that these hormones are something different than the hormones a health care provider might prescribe from a traditional pharmacy. However, they aren't. Most of the hormones I prescribe are also made in a lab and the intent is that they mimic the hormones your body previously created. Therefore, the estrogen patch I prescribe regularly is also a "bio-identical." However, the hormone treatments made in a compounding pharmacy are not regulated strictly like what we might get from an FDA-regulated pharmacy. I still use compounding pharmacies when I can't get things from a traditional pharmacy, like combined estrogen and testosterone creams for vaginal use, for example. But if I can get something prescribed by a regulated pharmacy and my patient can get insurance coverage for it, that is my preference.

Question to Consider:

1. How do you feel about hormones?
   a. I have a strong family history of breast cancer, so I don't touch them.
   b. I see the benefit and use some as needed.
   c. I've got a different hormonal treatment for each day of the week.

She told me, "Look, I have a younger boyfriend. I need to keep up." She was referring to her looks and to her sexual function and I empathized with her.

"Ok, let's just scrap everything and start with one hormone at a time so we can figure out what is helping with what. And let's do a baseline testosterone level since increasing sex drive is one of our main goals," I told her.

Not surprisingly, despite all the compounded testosterone and testosterone precursors she was using, her testosterone level was zero. She was spending hundreds if not thousands of dollars on creams and treatments that her body was not able to metabolize.

Why do these kinds of clinics exist? They are offering treatments that are not based on evidence or robust medical research findings. They exist because the North American healthcare system is failing women. My patients frequently tell me horror stories of being dismissed by their medical providers. They often feel rushed, not listened to, and many women do not feel comfortable bringing up these intimate aspects of their lives.

"Just drink some wine and relax!" is something many women have been told by my medical colleagues as maybe an "easy fix" statement, but really, it's damaging to women. There are bio-psycho-social reasons that we experience challenges with intimacy and it's best to approach treatment of these issues that way as well. There are many options for treatment with substantial research to back them up.

Positive affirmation: What I am experiencing is physiologic and connected to normal hormone changes. I do not have to suffer.

Chapter 10: After the Kids Fly the Coop – Let's Get Frisky!

Anna Myers

The tale of Jen and Ted is a riveting one; they've navigated through numerous relationship hurdles, triumphantly overcoming each one. Ted, initially struggling with maintaining an erection, found his saving grace in Cialis, and they ingeniously turned this challenge into a playful game. To signal her interest in a bit of intimacy later in the day, Jen would slyly slip a tablet into Ted's pocket before he headed off to work. This secret exchange became their amusing and anticipatory prelude to the passion that would unfold upon their reunion. Alas, the plot thickens as their youngest offspring, in the midst of a career switch, decides to move back in. With their newfound roommate, their afternoon trysts were abruptly halted.

They attempted to work around this by rescheduling their intimate moments, but exhaustion and the pressure to be discreet in front of their son dampened the mood. The spontaneity and excitement they once shared were replaced by stress and disappointment. "We're overthinking it. We just want our fun, carefree intimacy back," lamented Jen.

Yet, Jen and Ted had a good kind of problem. They had desire, had tackled all the physical aspects of their intimate relationship, and were only held back by their adult child's presence. Through various discussions, we brainstormed solutions such as monthly romantic getaways, weekly date nights, and strategically timed "alone time" on the nights their son hit the gym.

However, another issue many of my patients come in upset about is reconnecting with their partner after their children grow up. They may start grieving this impending change years in advance. Women often find themselves grappling with their changing bodies, relationships, and roles all at once during the menopause transition.

It's crucial to show yourself grace, recognizing that empty nesting is a significant life transition. However, it's also a golden opportunity for couples to rediscover each other and their relationship.

Apparently, "empty nest syndrome," this idea of crisis identity for parents, particularly mothers, was coined in the 1970s by sociologists, but research hasn't proven its accuracy. Empty nest depression and loss of purpose is a myth to debunk along with many others we have discussed in this book! Many people find this as a time of increased satisfaction and improved relationships not only with their partners but even other family members such as their siblings (Clay, 2003).

So what can we do? When I was on the verge of my children growing up and leaving me, I was fortunate to have a group of ladies at my church that took me aside and offered invaluable advice, helping me see this next life phase in a positive light. "Hey, you are going to love this next phase as much as the last because of the role you will still play in your children's lives. You will still be their parents and talk out the big stuff, staying part of their lives. But you won't have to deal with the day to day stuff; the laundry, the meals, etc. You know, the annoying stuff."

Research published in Psychological Medicine backs this up. For the majority of women, the last child leaving the household leads to positive moods and reduced number of daily hassles (Dennerstein et al. 2002).

I remember one friend pulled me aside and said, "You will enjoy it so much that when the kids come home it will actually put a cramp in your style…you'll almost feel a little put out as you'll have to start wearing your underwear again and cooking, etc."

My friends were right and armed with this insight, I made a mental decision to look at these years differently and embrace it. Were there times I thought about my girls and wanted to go visit them at school or bring them home when they had a bad day? Of course, but I could pick up the phone and call them on my way home from work. It felt good to still be the one they wanted to tell about their days.

Not only did I develop this new relationship with young adults whom I was very proud of, I got the opportunity to develop a deeper relationship with the partner who helped create this life we live together. In an investigation of women's marital satisfaction over 18 years of midlife, Gorchoff et.al. showed that women who made the transition to empty nest were more satisfied with their marriage than women with children at home (2008). They found that the empty nest doesn't increase marital satisfaction just because you have more time together but that women who had transitioned to the empty nest genuinely enjoyed the quality of the time spent with their partners more.

For us, it became a time to dream bigger than ever before. Watching a documentary, I was struck by a common theme among successful leaders reflecting on their past: the importance of dreaming big. The interviewers asked the leaders, "What would you tell your former self twenty years ago?" Nearly everyone answered with the same theme, "Dream big and bigger than you would have."

Start dreaming and planning on a regular basis. Make plans to try the things you want to try, go to the places you always said you'd love to go, try out whatever activity, live wherever, connect with old friends, or make new relationships. People who live long happy lives have something more important than physique, vaccinations, and healthy habits in common, they make social connections. Now is the time to catch up on all those lunch dates you put off while raising the kids.

Write a book, try a new hobby, a new job. I can't tell you how many patients come in to see me in their 70s, disappointed that they waited until retirement to do the things they wanted to try or places they wanted to travel as maybe their health or their partner's health didn't last or maybe they got busy with grandkids, elderly parents, or something else got in the way. I also have patients that say, "I lived an exciting life, we traveled while we worked, we started new hobbies, our own business, and my partner and I have the kids over regularly for parties."

So, as you navigate this new chapter, consider these techniques for reconnecting:

Communication: Open up about your feelings, desires, and expectations. Get into your partner's mind and learn where they are coming from. It will help with understanding and developing a deeper connection.

Shared Interests: Discover activities you both enjoy. From cooking to taking a dance class, shared interests strengthen that bond and you will create new memories together.

Date nights: This is the fun stuff! You might have more time at home with your partner, but you still need dating to keep the romance alive. Be spontaneous. If you don't feel like cooking, go to the local pub, listen to music on a weeknight! Make the date about trying new activities you never had the desire to try before together. Just the shared experience will be good for your relationship as you build this life post-children and make new memories of just the two of you. I remember that first winter after the kids moved out; we tried cross-country skiing. We won't likely do it again, but we have fond memories laughing as we saw 6-year-olds zoom past us while we slid off the path and had to help each other up. We eventually carried our skis at the end when we gave up and decided hot cocoa around the fire pit looked like more fun! Creating new hobbies helps to provide differentiation as well as an opportunity to fantasize about the partner and experience.

Travel: Traveling together can be a great way to reconnect and rediscover your relationship. Planning a romantic getaway or taking a trip to a new destination, helps you create new experiences and lasting memories.

Couples Counseling: If you're struggling, don't hesitate to seek professional help. A trained therapist can help you work through issues or conflicts and develop new strategies for strengthening a relationship.

Questions to Consider:

1. How do you currently feel about the prospect of an empty nest?
    a. I can't wait to have some time to myself. I'm sick of cooking and cleaning!
    b. I am worried that my partner and I have become strangers.
    c. I don't know what to expect. We may realize we grew further apart than we can recover from.

2. Dream. Do you have any personal goals or hobbies that you have been pondering or maybe

put aside while raising the kids that now would be a great time to bring to life?

a. Nope, I was so busy raising kids and working, I didn't have time to develop any personal hobbies or interests of my own.

b. I have so many friends to catch up with now that our kids have gone on to college this fall, we'll be able to have that weekly wine night or coffee date we kept planning on doing.

c. I'm open to new adventures! I'm planning a European vacation when my junior leaves for college in the fall!

3. What are some date nights or leisure activities you can list that you would like to consider with your partner?

a. _____

b. _____

c. _____

Affirmation: Our relationship is filled with trust, honesty, open communication, mutual understanding, shared experiences, and most of all love!

References:

Clay, RA. An empty nest can promote freedom, improved relationships: A developing line of research suggests that many parents get a new lease on life when their children leave. American Psychological Association. 2003 Apr; 34(4). Print version page 40. An empty nest can promote freedom, improved relationships (apa.org)

Dennerstein L, Dudley E, Guthrie J. Empty nest or revolving door? A prospective study of women's quality of life in midlife during the phase of children leaving and re-entering the home. Psychol Med. 2002 Apr;32(3):545-50. doi: 10.1017/s0033291701004810. PMID: 11989999.

Gorchoff, S. M., John, O. P., & Helson, R. (2008). Contextualizing change in marital satisfaction during middle age: An 18-year longitudinal study. *Psychological Science, 19*(11), 1194–1200. https://doi.org/10.1111/j.1467-9280.2008.02222.x

Appendix:

Sex, Drugs, and Rock-N-Roll:

Medications That Can Negatively Affect Your Sexual Health

It has been said that the brain is the largest sex organ which may be due to the interplay of various neurotransmitters within the brain. Dopamine, oxytocin, melanocortin, and norepinephrine stimulate a person's appetite for sex. Meanwhile, serotonin, opioids, endocannabinoids, and prolactin decrease a person's appetite for sex. Therefore, medications that increase the inhibitory neurotransmitters can also decrease a person's sex drive such as: selective serotonin reuptake inhibitors (SSRIs) and serotonin and norepinephrine reuptake inhibitors (SNRIs) both of which are often used to treat anxiety or depression.

Testosterone is an important hormone for women's sexual health including sex drive, orgasm, arousal and lubrication. Medications that decrease testosterone and therefore can negatively affect sexual health include oral combined (both estrogen and progesterone) birth control pills or spironolactone.

Alcohol may decrease inhibition but can also cause vaginal dryness due to dehydration and decrease sensation in women. (It can cause delayed orgasm in men.)

Beta-blockers are prescribed to treat both high blood pressure and irregular heart rhythms but they may cause a decrease in arousal and orgasm in men and women.

Estrogen is also an important hormone for women's sexual health. It is important for lubrication, arousal, and orgasm. However, aromatase inhibitors (AIs) used in breast cancer treatment significantly decrease the amount of circulating estrogen.

Although the above listed medications can negatively influence sexual health, their benefits may still outweigh these risks. Discuss any concerns with your health care provider including if there are alternative options.

Book Club: some of our favorite books that you may also enjoy

1.   **Broken Open:** How Difficult Times Can Help Us Grow: by Elizabeth Lesser

Great book when you need some reassurance that you are not alone in your struggles and has great coping techniques.

2.   **Rekindling Desire:** by Barry and Emily McCarthy

How to keep the romance and desire going in long-term relationships.

3.   **Come as You Are:** by Emily Nagoski

Everything women should know about sex and their bodies.

4.   **The Book of Joy:** Lasting Happiness in a Changing World: by the 14th Dalai Lama and Archbishop Desmond Tutu

This book changed my life and how I live it-Jean.

5.   **Sex in Your Sixties:** by Jean Marino, Rachel Pope, Anna Myers, Karen Connor, Erika Kelly, and Sheryl Kingsberg

We collaborated with our women's sexual health colleagues to write this book.

6. **Becoming Cliterate**: by Laurie Mintz

Dr. Mintz makes the argument that the #1 reason for orgasm disparity is by the assumption that women are supposed to reach climax through penetration alone.

Websites:

The Menopause Retreat;
www.menopauseandsexualhealth.com

The Menopause Society;
www.menopause.org

www.OMGYES.com

A letter to my Partner/Loved One:

I am going through the transition of menopause, and I could use your support. I know it's tough to understand what I'm feeling and experiencing, but I thought of an idea. Try to remember back to when you started going through puberty. Maybe you were 13 or 14. You started finding hair growing where it hadn't before, your body started changing, your moods probably changed a bit, and you might have felt like you didn't have control over it all. Everyone around you started to notice and sometimes those interactions were uncomfortable! Relatives would insensitively comment, "Wow, you've lost your baby weight now that you're so tall!" or "Have you considered Accutane?"

Some changes were probably positive, but some were also inconvenient. The hardest part is that you didn't know exactly where the changes would end and what the new normal would be. On top of that, you might not have had anyone to talk to about it in a non-judgmental way.

This is a lot of what I'm going through right now with mood changes that I can't explain, sleep changes, body changes, etc. Sometimes my hot flashes or night sweats are so bad that I don't feel well rested the next day. Sometimes my brain fog is so difficult I'm nervous that I have early onset Alzheimer's. My body is not responding to the exercise and healthy eating it used to and I feel self-conscious at times. Sometimes I don't really feel sexy, and when I do convince myself to "get over it," sometimes intercourse can be painful in ways it never used to be. These are all things that might be happening now or in the near future and I just want to let you know so that you know I am still me on the inside, and I would love to have your support while I get through it.

I am grateful to have a community of other women going through the same things, which is why you might find me attending meetings and joining online groups. Most of all, I need your support while I go through this transition. Please don't be offended if I snap at you and please feel free to give me a comforting hug if it looks like I need one.

Your support and love means everything to me. Thank you for taking the time to try to understand.

Love,

Me

.

.

www.ingramcontent.com/pod-product-compliance
Lightning Source LLC
Chambersburg PA
CBHW070320290526
45791CB00003B/1189